MW01230622

Mediterranean Diet Recipe Book

Effortless and Foolproof Recipes to Embrace Lifelong Health

Asher Nelson

Legal & Disclaimer

The information contained in this book and its contents is not designed to replace or take the place of any form of medical or professional advice; and is not meant to replace the need for independent medical, financial, legal or other professional advice or services, as may be required. The content and information in this book has been provided for educational and entertainment purposes only.

The content and information contained in this book has been compiled from sources deemed reliable, and it is accurate to the best of the Author's knowledge, information and belief. However, the Author cannot guarantee its accuracy and validity and cannot be held liable for any errors and/or omissions. Further, changes are periodically made to this book as and when needed. Where appropriate and/or necessary, you must consult a professional (including but not limited to your doctor, attorney, financial advisor or such other professional advisor) before using any of the suggested remedies, techniques, or information in this book.

Upon using the contents and information contained in this book, you agree to hold harmless the Author from and against any damages, costs, and expenses, including any legal fees potentially resulting from the application of any of the information provided by this book.

Table of Contents

Introduction

The Mediterranean diet is one of the most effective ways to lose weight and prevent heart disease. The Mediterranean diet is great for your skin because it's full of antioxidants. It also contains plenty of fresh fruit and vegetables, which are packed with vitamins and minerals that can help to protect the skin from free radicals and inflammation. The Mediterranean diet has been proven to be one of the healthiest diets around. The diet is low in saturated fat and high in complex carbohydrates, such as fruits, vegetables, nuts and whole grains.

The Mediterranean diet is a healthy eating plan that has been proven in numerous studies to prevent heart disease, lower the risk of cancer, and even slow down the aging process. The Mediterranean diet is a good healthy diet that's full of fruits and vegetables, nuts, seeds, fish, olives and olive oil. It has been shown to reduce the risk of heart disease and several cancers. The Mediterranean diet includes a healthy diet of fruits, vegetables, whole grains, fish and olive oil. It's important to have a variety of foods in your diet as part of a balanced meal plan.

A Mediterranean diet is a great way to ensure you're getting all the essential nutrients and micronutrients you need. It includes things like fresh fruit, vegetables, whole grains and lean sources of protein. The Mediterranean diet is one of the healthiest diets in the world and has some great benefits for both your health and skin. The advantages of the Mediterranean diet include better heart health, lower risk of diabetes, cancer and Alzheimer's disease. This is because it is low in saturated fat and high in fresh fruit and vegetables.

The Mediterranean diet is a diet that is rich in healthy fats, lean protein, fruits and vegetables. It's high in antioxidants and has been shown to improve heart health and reduce the risk of chronic disease. According to the Mediterranean Diet Pyramid, research shows that this diet can improve your overall health and wellbeing. It's high in fiber, antioxidants, and healthy fats from olive oil and fish. The Mediterranean diet is a great diet because it's simple and easy to follow, but the benefits are huge. It's rich in fruits, vegetables, whole grains, and fish and it prevents you from getting heart disease or cancer.

The Mediterranean diet, also known as the 'Mediterranean way of eating,' is a lifestyle that combines elements of three traditional Mediterranean food cultures: the Greek, the Italian and the Provencal. The Mediterranean diet is rich with variety, and includes lots of fresh produce, healthy oils, unprocessed meat, fish and cheese. This diet has been shown to help reduce the risk of heart disease, type 2 diabetes and some types of cancer. One of the great things about the Mediterranean diet is that it's based on whole grains, vegetables, fruit, and lean proteins. These foods are great for your health and will help you lose weight.

This is a diet that is based on whole foods with an emphasis on plant-based foods like vegetables, fruit, whole grains, and nuts. The idea is to focus on what you're eating instead of focusing on calories or fat. The Mediterranean diet has a lot of health benefits, but it's also been linked to better brain function. The Mediterranean diet is one of the most researched and tested diets in the world.

Breakfast

1. Mediterranean Frittata

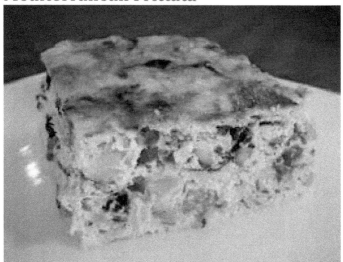

Preparation Time: 5 minutes

Cooking Time: 25 minutes

Servings: 2

Ingredients:

- Eggs, six
- Black pepper, one-quarter of a teaspoon
- Milk, one-quarter of a cup
- Oregano, one teaspoon
- Tomatoes, one-quarter of a cup, diced
- Salt, one teaspoon
- Green olives, one-quarter of a cup, chopped finely
- Feta cheese, one-quarter of a cup, crumble

- Black olives, one-quarter of a cup, chopped finely

Directions:

Heat the oven to 400. Spray oil an eight-by-eight-inch baking dish. Beat the milk into the eggs, and then add the other ingredients. Pour this mixture into the baking dish and bake for twenty minutes.

Nutrition:

Calories 107

7 grams fat

705 milligrams sodium

3 grams carbs

2 grams sugars

7 grams protein

2. Mediterranean Eggs

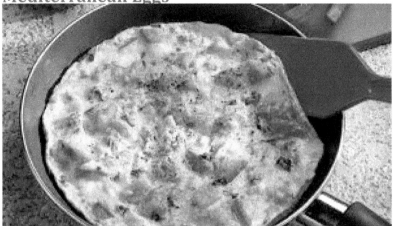

Preparation Time: 5 minutes

Cooking Time: 1 hour and 18 minutes

Servings: 2

Ingredients:

- Yellow onion, one large, cut in thin slices
- Parsley, one-quarter of a cup, chopped finely
- Butter, one tablespoon
- Sea salt, one-quarter of a teaspoon
- Olive oil, one tablespoon
- Black pepper, one-half of a teaspoon
- Garlic, one clove, chopped fine
- Feta cheese, three ounces, crumbled small
- Tomatoes, one-half of a cup, cut in thin slices
- Eggs, eight

Directions:

Cook the onions in the butter until they are soft for about ten minutes.

Stir in the olive oil, along with the tomatoes and garlic and cook for five more minutes.

Lower the heat and break the eggs over the mix, drizzling with pepper, salt, and feta.

Cover and cook for ten minutes without stirring over low heat.

Sprinkle on the parsley and serve.

Nutrition:

Calories 183

11 grams carbs

9 grams protein

11 grams fat

255 milligrams sodium

1 gram fiber

6 grams sugar

3. Southwest Tofu Scramble

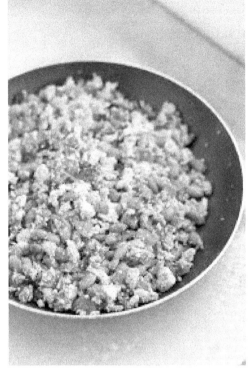

Preparation Time: 10 minutes

Cooking Time: 20 minutes

Servings: 2

Ingredients:

- Kale, two cups, washed, dried, and chopped into small pieces
- Eggs, four, beaten well
- Red pepper, one-half of one, sliced thinly
- Olive oil, two tablespoons
- Red onion, one-fourth of one, sliced thinly

- Garlic powder, one teaspoon
- Turmeric, a quarter teaspoon
- Water, just enough to thin ingredients
- Chili powder, a quarter teaspoon
- Sea salt, one-half teaspoon
- Cumin powder, one-half teaspoon

Directions:

To make the sauce, mix all of the spices together in a bowl, and add just enough water to stir into a sauce-type of consistency.

Cook the red pepper, kale, and onion for three to four minutes in the olive oil.

Then pour the beaten egg all over the mix in the pan, and cook it until the eggs reach your desired set.

Nutrition:

Calories 252

19 grams fat

516 milligrams sodium

12.7 grams carbs

3 grams fiber

2.5 grams sugar

12 grams protein

4. Mediterranean Breakfast Salad

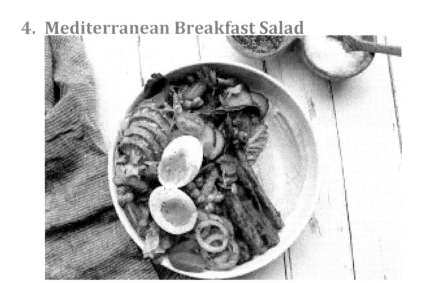

Preparation Time: 30 minutes

Cooking Time: 0 minutes

Servings: 2

Ingredients:

- Eggs, four, hard-boiled and sliced in thin slices
- Lemon juice, three tablespoons
- Arugula, ten cups, washed and d ried
- Olive oil, two tablespoons
- Tomato, one large, cut into eight wedges
- Dill, one-half of a cup, chopped finely
- Cucumber, one-half of a cup, chopped finely
- Almonds, one cup, chopped finely
- Quinoa, one cup, cooked and already cooled
- Avocado, one large, sliced in thin slices

Directions:

Mix the quinoa with the tomatoes, cucumber, and arugula.

Add the salt, pepper, and olive oil; toss lightly.

Place the salad mix on four salad plates, arrange the sliced egg and the avocado slices on top of the salad mix, and top with the almonds and herbs.

Drizzle the lemon juice all over it.

Nutrition:

Calories 336

7.7 grams fat

946.4 milligrams sodium

54.6 grams carbs

5.2 grams fiber

5.5 grams sugar

12.3 grams protein

5. Gingerbread Banana Bake with Quinoa

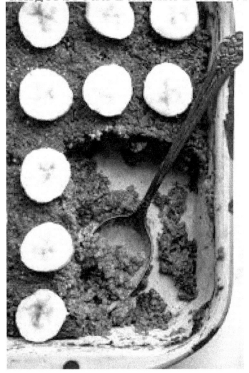

Preparation Time: 10 minutes

Cooking Time: 1 hour and 20 minutes

Servings: 2

Ingredients:

- Bananas, three cups, mashed
- Almonds, slivered, one-quarter cup
- Cinnamon, one tablespoon
- Milk, two and one-half cups
- Ginger, one teaspoon ginger

- Quinoa, one cup
- Salt, one-half teaspoon
- Allspice, one-half teaspoon, ground
- Cloves, one teaspoon, ground

Directions:

Heat the oven to 350.

Use oil spray on a nine by thirteen baking dish. Blend together the salt, vanilla, cloves, ginger, allspice, cinnamon, and bananas until smooth.

Stir in the milk and quinoa.

Pour this mixture into a baking dish and bake covered for one hour. After this, take it out of the oven and uncover.

Drizzle on sliced almonds and bake for another twenty minutes.

Nutrition:

Calories 213

4 grams fat

41 grams carbs

18 grams sugar

211 milligrams sodium

4 grams fiber

5 grams protein

6. Avocado and Feta Cheese Baked Eggs

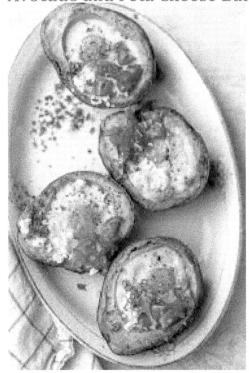

Preparation Time: 25 minutes

Cooking Time: 15 minutes

Servings: 2

Ingredients:

- Salt and pepper, one-quarter of a teaspoon each
- Eggs, four
- Feta cheese, three tablespoons, crumbled finely
- Avocado, one large, cut into slices
- Olive oil, two tablespoons

Directions:

Heat the oven to 350. Lay the slices of avocado into two oven-safe personal-sized baking dishes.

Crack two of the eggs into each bowl easily, so you do not break the yoke.

Add the cheese crumbles and lightly sprinkle pepper and salt in each cup. Bake them for fifteen minutes.

Nutrition:

Calories 329

2.2 grams carbs

17 grams protein

7. Santa Fe Taco Salad

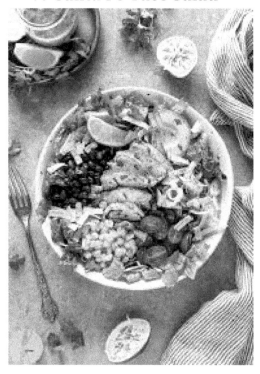

Preparation Time: 11 minutes

Cooking Time: 16 minutes

Servings: 2

Ingredients

Toppings:

- ½ pound 93 percent lean ground turkey (1 lean)
- 1/2 cup dried, rinsed, and drained black beans (1/2 healthy fat)

- Seasoned jalapeño chili pepper (1/4 green)
- Beefsteak tomatoes, chopped (1/2 healthy fat)
- 1 Clove of garlic, minced and peeled (1/8 condiment)
- 3 tablespoons of chopped scallions (1/2 green)
- 2 tablespoons of fresh cilantro chopped, plus garnish (1/2 green)
- Salt and ground black pepper, sweet paprika to taste 1 ¼ teaspoon (1/8 condiment)

For the Avocado Dip:

- ¼ cup, 2% Greek yogurt (1/2 healthy fat)
- ¼ cup of water (1/2 condiment)
- 1 medium avocado, peeled, pitted, chopped, and split (1/2 healthy fat)
- 1 ½ spoonful of fresh cilantro (1/4 green)
- ½ tablespoon cayenne pepper (1/8 condiment)
- Salt and black chili pepper, to taste (1/8 condiment)

For the Salad:

- 5 cups shredded iceberg lettuce cup shredded (1 green)
- 1 Mexican cheese mixed beefsteak tomato, chopped (1/2 healthy fat)
- Tablespoons of fresh coriander (1/2 green)
- 2 spoons smashed tortilla chips (1/2 healthy fat)

Directions:

Heat a broad skillet over medium-high heat, without sticking. Use a wooden spoon to split the meat into small pieces and add the ground turkey to the skillet. Cook, stirring constantly, for 4 to 5 minutes until the meat is no longer pink.

Incorporate beans, jalapeño, onions, garlic, scallions, salt, pepper, and paprika. Reduce heat to low, cover, and cook for 15 minutes. Remove the lid from the skillet and cook for about 5 minutes until the liquid decreases.

In the meantime, make the avocado dip: add yogurt, sugar, half the avocado, cilantro, cayenne, salt, and pepper into a blender. Up to a smooth process; reserve.

Divide the lettuce into 4 slabs. Top with the mixture of beef, cheese, onions, cilantro, and chopped avocado left over. Add the avocado dip over the top and garnish the chips with crushed tortilla.

Nutrition:

491 calories

28g fat

11g protein

8. Mushroom and Spinach Omelet

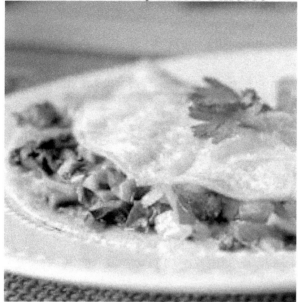

Preparation Time: 3 minutes

Cooking Time: 15 minutes

Servings: 2

Ingredients:

- Olive oil, one tablespoon
- Green onion, one, diced finely
- Red onion, one-quarter of a cup, diced finely
- Egg, three
- Spinach, one and one-half fresh, chopped small
- Feta cheese, one-half of a cup, crumbled small
- Button mushrooms, five, sliced thinly

Directions:

Sauté the onions, mushrooms, and spinach for three minutes in the olive oil and then set them to the side.

Pour the well-beaten eggs into the skillet.

Let the eggs cook for three to four minutes until the edges begin to brown.

Sprinkle all of the other ingredients onto half of the omelet and then fold the other half over the ingredients.

Cook the omelet for one minute on each side.

Nutrition:

Calories 337

25 grams fat

911 milligrams sodium

5.4 grams carbs

1 gram fiber

1.3 grams sugar

22 grams protein

9. Fruit Bulgur

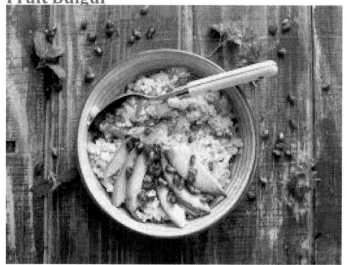

Preparation Time: 5 minutes

Cooking Time: 10 minutes

Servings: 2

Ingredients:

- 2 Cups Milk, 2%
- 1 ½ Cups Bulgur, Uncooked
- ½ Teaspoon Cinnamon
- 2 Cups Dark Sweet cherries, Frozen
- 8 Figs, Dried & Chopped
- ½ Cup Almonds, Chopped
- ¼ Cup Mint, Fresh & Chopped
- ½ Cup Almonds, Chopped
- Warm 2% Milk to Serve

Directions:

Get out a medium saucepan and combine your water, cinnamon, bulgur and milk together.

Stir it once and bring it just to a boil. Once it begins to boil then cover it, and then reduce your heat to medium-low. Allow it to simmer for ten minutes. The liquid should be absorbed.

Turn the heat off, but keep your pan on the stove. Stir in your frozen cherries. You don't need to thaw them, and then ad din your almonds and figs. Stir well before covering for a minute.

Stir your mint in, and then serve with warm milk drizzled over it.

Nutrition:

Calories: 301

Protein: 9 Grams

Fat: 6 Grams

Carbs: 57 Grams

Sodium: 40 mg

10.   Mediterranean Toast

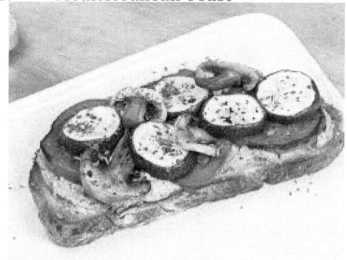

Preparation Time: 10 minutes

Cooking Time: 5 minutes

Servings: 2

Ingredients:

- 1 Slice Whole Wheat Bread
- 1 Tablespoon Roasted Red Pepper Hummus
- 3 Cherry Tomatoes, Sliced
- ¼ Avocado, Mashed
- 3 Greek Olives, Sliced
- 1 Hardboiled Egg, Sliced
- 1 ½ Teaspoons Crumbled Feta Cheese, Reduced Fat

Directions:

Start by topping your toast with ¼ avocado and then your hummus.

Add your remaining ingredients and season with salt and pepper before serving.

Nutrition:

Calories: 314

Protein: 4.2 Grams

Fat: 28.7 Grams

Carbs: 13.2 Grams

Sodium: 84 mg

11.   Goat Cheese & Pepper Eggs

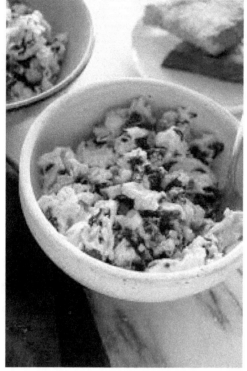

Preparation Time: 5 minutes

Cooking Time: 5 minutes

Servings: 2

Ingredients:

- 1 Cup Bell Pepper, Chopped
- 1 ½ Teaspoons Olive Oil
- 2 Cloves Garlic, Minced
- 6 Eggs, Large
- ¼ Teaspoon Sea Salt, Fine

- 2 Tablespoons Water
- ½ Cup Goat Cheese, Crumbled
- 2 Tablespoons Mint, fresh & chopped

Directions:

Start by getting a large skillet out and placing it over medium-high heat. Add in your oil. Once your oil begins to shimmer add in your peppers and allow them to cook for five minutes. Stir occasionally, and then add in your garlic and cook a minute more.

While your peppers cook whisk your slat, water and eggs together. Turn the heat to medium-low. Pour your egg mixture over the peppers, and then let them cook for about two minutes without stirring them. They should set on the bottom before you sprinkle your goat cheese over top.

Cook your eggs for another two minutes, and then serve with fresh mint.

Nutrition:

Calories: 201

Protein: 15 Grams

Fat: 15 Grams

Carbs: 5 Grams

Sodium: 166 mg

12.   Mediterranean Egg Cups

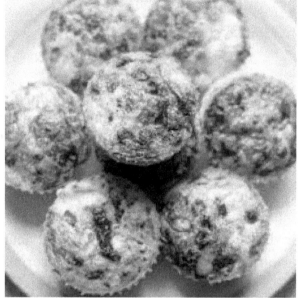

Preparation Time: 15 minutes

Cooking Time: 25 minutes

Servings: 2

Ingredients:

- Bell pepper, one cup chopped finely
- Feta cheese, three tablespoons crumbled small
- Mushrooms, one cup chopped finely
- Eggs, ten
- Black pepper, one-quarter of a teaspoon
- Milk, two-thirds of a cup
- Salt, one-quarter of a teaspoon
- Garlic powder, one teaspoon

- Spray oil

Directions:

Heat the oven to 350. Spray oil in the twelve-muffin cup pan. Add the pepper, salt, garlic powder, and milk into the beaten egg until mixed well.

Add in the peppers and the mushrooms.

Fill the muffin pan cups with this mix. Bake for twenty-five minutes. Cool for five minutes then top with the cheese and serve.

Nutrition:

Calories 67

4.7 grams fat

Sodium 161.4 milligrams

1.2 grams carbs

.7 grams sugar

4.6 grams protein

13.   Breakfast Egg on Avocado

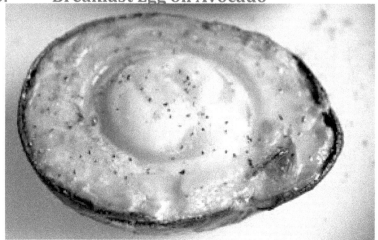

Preparation Time: 10 minutes

Cooking Time: 15 minutes

Servings: 2

Ingredients:

- 1 tsp. garlic powder
- 1/2 tsp. sea salt
- 1/4 cup Parmesan cheese (grated or shredded)
- 1/4 tsp. black pepper
- 3 medium avocados (cut in half, pitted, skin on)
- 6 medium eggs

Directions:

Prepare muffin tins and preheat the oven to 350oF.

To ensure that the egg would fit inside the cavity of the avocado, lightly scrape off 1/3 of the meat.

Place avocado on muffin tin to ensure that it faces with the top up.

Evenly season each avocado with pepper, salt, and garlic powder.

Add one egg on each avocado cavity and garnish tops with cheese.

Pop in the oven and bake until the egg white is set, about 15 minutes.

Serve and enjoy.

Nutrition:

Calories per serving: 252

Protein: 14.0g

Carbs: 4.0g

Fat: 20.0g

14.   Multigrain Blueberry Yogurt Pancakes

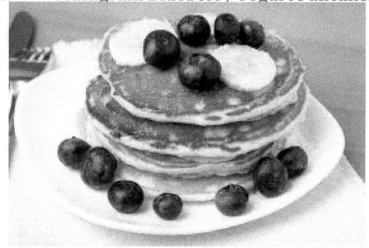

Preparation Time: 10 minutes

Cooking Time: 20 minutes

Servings: 2

Ingredients:

- Blueberries, one cup, fresh
- Eggs, two
- Salt, one-quarter teaspoon
- Plain Greek yogurt, one cup
- Baking powder, one teaspoon and one tablespoon
- Milk, four tablespoons
- Barley or rye flour, one-quarter of a cup
- All-purpose flour, one-half of a cup
- Butter, three tablespoons, melted
- Wheat flour, one-half of a cup

- Lemon zest, one teaspoon
- Vanilla, one teaspoon

Directions:

Blend together the milk, eggs, yogurt, and butter.

Mix the dry ingredients together in a separate bowl.

Spoon the wet ingredients gently into the dry ingredients and blend.

Pour the batter, one-quarter of a cup for each pancake, into the hot skillet that has been oiled with a light coating of olive oil.

Cook each pancake for three to four minutes on each side.

Nutrition:

Calories 98

3.2 grams fat

141 milligrams sodium

15 grams carbs

1.7 grams fiber

1.7 grams sugar

3.1 grams protein

15.   Classic Shakshouka-Style Mediterranean Breakfast

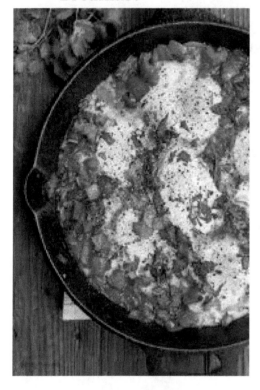

Preparation Time: 10 minutes

Cooking Time: 20 minutes

Servings: 2

Ingredients:

- Parsley, one tablespoon, chopped finely
- Eggs, four
- Olive oil, two tablespoons

- Chili sauce any variety, one teaspoon
- Black pepper, one teaspoon
- Tomatoes, two cups, chopped
- Salt, one-half of one teaspoon
- Garlic, two cloves, chopped finely
- Onion, one large yellow, shredded thinly
- Red bell peppers, two, shredded thinly

Directions:

Cook the garlic, peppers, and onions for five minutes in the olive oil.

Mix in the chili sauce and the tomatoes; cook for five more minutes.

Sprinkle in the pepper and salt.

Make four round spaces in the mix in the pan, and break the eggs gently into the spaces.

Cook for five minutes until the eggs are set.

Nutrition:

Calories 304; 18.1 grams fat; 623 milligrams sodium; 23.1 grams carbs; 3.8 grams fiber; 1.2 grams sugar; 14.3 grams protein

Lunch

16.   Creamy Rice Risotto with Mushrooms and Thyme

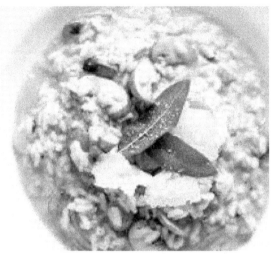

Preparation Time: 20 minutes

Cooking Time: 15 minutes

Servings: 2

Ingredients:

- 2 Tbsp. olive oil
- 1 onion, finely chopped
- 4 garlic cloves, finely chopped
- 13 oz. Arborio rice
- 4 cups sliced mushrooms (use any type!)
- ½ cup dry white wine

- 2 Tbsp. thyme leaves, finely chopped
- 6 ½ cups vegetable or chicken stock
- 3 Tbsp. butter
- ½ cup grated parmesan cheese
- Salt and pepper

Directions:

Place the stock into a saucepan over a medium heat, it shouldn't boil, but should be hot and steaming

Add the olive oil to a large sauté pan or pot over a medium heat

Add the rice and stir to coat in olive oil, allow the rice to become acquainted with the flavor of the onion and garlic, about 3 minutes

Add the mushrooms and stir as they soften for about 3 minutes

Add zucchinis the onion and garlic and stir as they soften and become fragrant, about 3 minutes

the wine and stir to deglaze the corners of the pan, allow it to reduce for about 3 minutes

Add the thyme leaves and stir

Add a dash of hot stock, stir, and allow it to be absorbed into the rice. Repeat this process, adding dashes of hot stock, stirring, and allowing to absorb, until all of the stock has been used up and the risotto is creamy

Stir the butter, parmesan, salt and pepper into the risotto, cover, and leave for at least 5 minutes. This step is crucial for a creamy risotto!

The butter and cheese melt, and the starches from the rice have time to relax and create a silky, rich consistency

Serve with a little extra sprinkle of grated parmesan and a few thyme leaves!

Nutrition:

Calories: 608

Fat: 19.4 grams

Protein: 23.2 grams

Total carbs: 80.3 grams

Net carbs: 79.8 grams

17.   Pearl Barley, Citrus, and Broccoli Salad

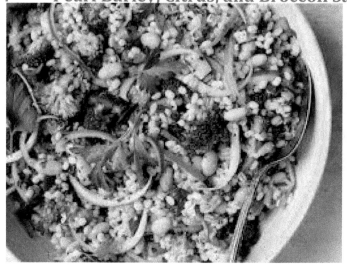

Preparation Time: 25 minutes

Cooking Time: 20 minutes

Servings: 2

Ingredients:

- 1 ½ cups pearl barley
- 4 ¼ cups water
- Salt
- 2 oranges, peeled and chopped
- 1 medium-large head of broccoli, cut into florets
- 3 oz. feta cheese, crumbled
- 1/3 cup chopped almonds, gently toasted
- 1/3 cup chopped hazelnuts, gently toasted
- ½ cup finely chopped parsley

- 3 Tbsp. olive oil
- Salt and pepper

Directions:

Place the barley, water, and salt into a saucepan over a medium heat, cover, and bring to boiling point

Reduce to a simmer, and partially remove the cover

Keep an eye on the barley and add a dash of water if it appears to be drying out

When the barley is plump and there is no liquid left, remove the pot from the heat and allow the barley to cool a little

Place a steamer over a saucepan of shallow, boiling water, add the broccoli to the steamer, cover, and cook until the broccoli is just cooked but still crunchy and vibrant in color

Combine the pearl barley, broccoli, feta, almonds, hazelnuts, parsley, olive oil, salt and pepper in a salad bowl and toss to combine

Nutrition:

Calories: 569

Fat: 28.2 grams

Protein: 19.1 grams

Total carbs: 80 grams

Net carbs: 60 grams

18.   Beetroot and Goat Cheese Salad with Toasted Barley

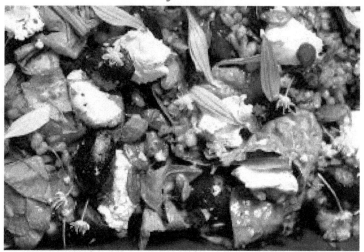

Preparation Time: 25 minutes

Cooking Time: 15 minutes

Servings: 2

Ingredients:

- 1 ½ cups pearl barley
- 4 ½ cups water
- Salt
- 1 Tbsp. olive oil
- 2 large fresh beets, peeled and cut into chunks
- 1 Tbsp. olive oil
- Fresh thyme
- 4 oz. goat cheese, crumbled

- 6 Tbsp. pumpkin seeds, lightly toasted
- 4 cups baby spinach leaves, roughly chopped
- Salt and pepper
- Juice of 1 lemon

Directions:

Preheat the oven to 400 degrees Fahrenheit and line a baking tray with baking paper

Lay the beets onto the tray, rub with olive oil, and sprinkle with salt, thyme leaves, and pepper and place into the oven to roast for about 30 minutes or until soft, turning halfway through

Place the barley, water, and salt into a saucepan over a medium heat, cover, and bring to boiling point. Reduce the heat and allow the barley to simmer until there's no liquid left, and the barley is chewy

Push the beets aside on the baking tray and spread the cooked barley onto the tray and slip into the oven to toast for about 15 minutes (if you're worried about overcooking the beets you can transfer them into a salad bowl at this point)

In a salad bowl, toss together the beets, barley, goat cheese, spinach, pumpkin seeds, salt, pepper, and lemon juice

Serve warm or cold

Nutrition:

Calories: 506

Fat: 21.7 grams

Protein: 18.4 grams

Total carbs: 63.8 grams

Net carbs: 50 grams

19. Brown Lentil Salad with Grilled Halloumi

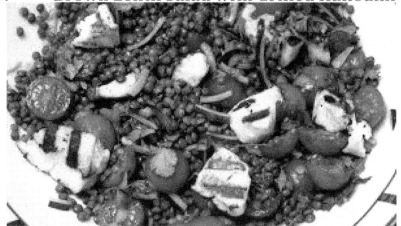

Preparation Time: 15 minutes

Cooking Time: 15 minutes

Servings: 2

Ingredients:

- 2 cans brown lentils (rinsed and drained)
- Juice and zest of 1 lemon
- 2 cups chopped cucumber (I leave the seeds in!)
- ½ cup toasted pine nuts (use almonds or cashews if pine nuts are too expensive in your region)
- 2 Tbsp. olive oil
- 14 oz. halloumi cheese, cut into strips

Directions:

Preheat the oven to 450 degrees Fahrenheit and line a baking tray with baking paper

In a large salad bowl, toss together the lentils, lemon, cucumber, pine nuts, and olive oil, set aside or refrigerate as you cook the halloumi

Place the halloumi slices onto the lined tray and cook in the upper third of the oven for about 12 minutes, turn the slices over, and cook until the other side is golden

Serve the salad with halloumi slices on top

Nutrition:

Calories: 665

Fat: 43.7 grams

Protein: 38 grams

Total carbs: 36.7 grams

Net carbs: 27.5 grams

20.   Israeli Couscous with Zucchini, Peas, and Feta

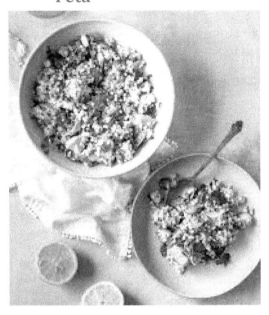

Preparation Time: 15 minutes

Cooking Time: 35 minutes

Servings: 2

Ingredients:

- 2 large zucchinis, cut into rounds
- 2 Tbsp. olive oil
- Salt and pepper
- Rosemary sprig
- 1 lemon, quartered
- 1 Tbsp. olive oil

- 1 Tbsp. butter
- 4 garlic cloves, roughly chopped
- 2 cups Israeli couscous (dry)
- 4 cups chicken or vegetable stock
- Salt and pepper
- 2 cups frozen peas, cooked (microwave, steam, or boil)
- 4 oz. feta cheese, crumbled

Directions:

Preheat the oven to 400 degrees Fahrenheit and line a baking tray with baking paper

Lay the zucchini rounds onto the tray, rub with olive oil, salt, and pepper. Nestle the rosemary and lemon quarters into the zucchini and slip into the oven to roast for about 30 minutes

While the zucchini is cooking, prepare the couscous: add the olive oil, butter, and garlic into a deep-sided sauté pan over a medium heat and allow the butter to melt and become frothy. Add the Israeli couscous, toss in the oil and butter, and toast for about 5 minutes. Add the stock, cover, and leave to cook until the stock has evaporated and the couscous is tender

Add the zucchini, peas, and feta to the pan with the couscous. Take the roasted lemon quarters and squeeze the gooey flesh and juices into the couscous and toss to combine

Serve warm or cold!

Nutrition: Calories: 610; Fat: 20 grams; Protein: 23.6 grams; Total carbs: 86.5 grams; Net carbs: 76.4 grams

21.   Artichokes Provencal

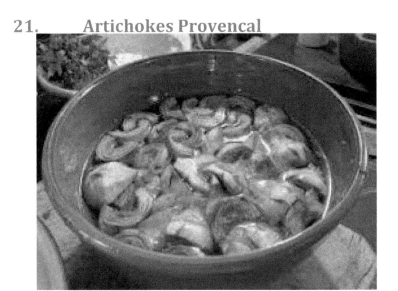

Preparation Time: 5 minutes

Cooking Time: 15 minutes

Servings: 2

Ingredients:

- 1 Tbsp. olive oil
- 1 onion, roughly chopped
- 4 garlic cloves, finely chopped
- ½ cup dry white wine
- 4 tomatoes, chopped
- 10 oz. artichoke hearts, quartered
- 1 lemon, quartered
- Salt and pepper
- Fresh basil, roughly chopped or torn

Directions:

Add the olive oil to a large sauté pan over a medium-high heat

Add the onions and garlic and stir as they soften, about 5 minutes

Add the wine and allow to reduce for a few minutes

Add the artichokes, tomatoes, salt, pepper, and lemon quarters, cover, and cook for about 5-8 minutes or until the artichokes are tender

Serve with fresh basil

Nutrition:

Calories: 159

Fat: 7 grams

Protein: 2.8 grams

Total carbs: 15.5 grams

Net carbs: 13.5 grams

22.   Bulgur and Roasted Bell Pepper Salad

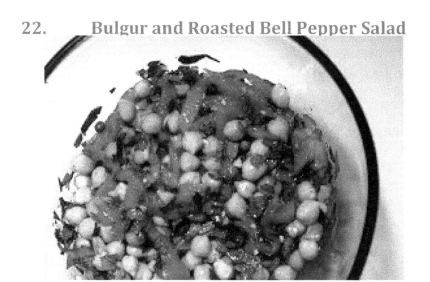

Preparation Time: 10 minutes

Cooking Time: 30 minutes

Servings: 2

Ingredients:

- 3 large red bell peppers, seeds removed, sliced
- 1 red onion, sliced
- 2 Tbsp. olive oil
- Salt and pepper
- 2 Tbsp. butter
- 1 Tbsp. olive oil
- 2 cups bulgur (dry)
- 4 cups water
- Salt

Directions:

Preheat the oven to 400 degrees Fahrenheit and line a baking tray with baking paper

Spread the bell pepper and onion over the tray and rub with olive oil, salt and pepper

Roast the bell pepper and onion for about 30 minutes, tossing once, until very soft and slightly charred and gooey

Add the butter and oil in a sauté pan over a medium heat

When the butter and oil are hot, add the dry bulgur and stir as it toasts, about 2 minutes

Add the water and salt to the pan, cover, and cook until the water has evaporated and the bulgur is fluffy and tender

Add the roasted bell pepper and onion to the bulgur, toss, and serve

Serving suggestions: fresh basil or mint and a side of lemony Greek yogurt

Nutrition:

Calories: 428

Fat: 17 grams

Protein: 10 grams

Total carbs: 63 grams

Net carbs: 51 grams

23.   Seafood Stuffing

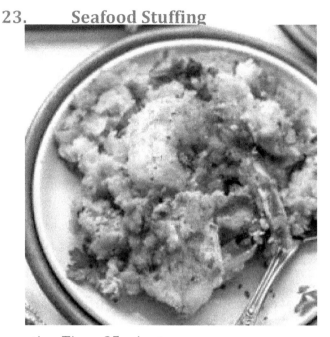

Preparation Time: 25 minutes

Cooking Time: 30 minutes

Servings: 2

Ingredients:

- 1/2 cup butter
- 1/2 cup chopped green pepper
- 1/2 cup chopped onion
- 1/2 cup chopped celery
- Drained and flaky crabmeat
- 1/2 pound of medium-sized shrimp - peeled and deveined
- 1/2 cup spiced and seasoned breadcrumbs
- 1 mixture of filling for cornbread

- 2 tablespoons of white sugar, divided
- 1 can of mushroom soup (10.75 ounces) condensed
- oz. chicken broth

Directions:

Melt the butter in a large frying pan over medium heat. Add pepper, onion, celery crabmeat and shrimp; boil and stir for about 5 minutes. Set aside.

In a large bowl, mix stuffing, breadcrumbs, and 1 tablespoon sugar. Stir the vegetables and seafood from the pan. Add the mushroom cream and as much chicken broth as you want. Pour into a 9 x 13-inch baking dish.

Bake in the preheated oven for 30 minutes or until lightly roasted.

Nutrition:

344 calories

15.7 grams of fat

28.4 g of carbohydrates

22 g of protein

94 mg of cholesterol

1141 mg of sodium

24.   Scrumptious Salmon Cakes

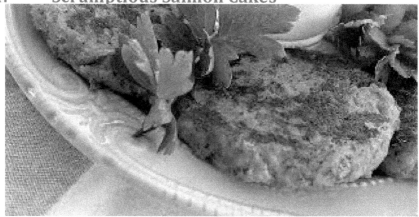

Preparation Time: 15 minutes

Cooking Time: 15 minutes

Servings: 2

Ingredients:

- 2 cans of salmon, drained and crumbled
- 3/4 cup Italian breadcrumbs
- 1/2 cup chopped fresh parsley
- 2 eggs, beaten
- 2 green onions, minced
- 2 teaspoons seafood herbs
- 1 1/2 teaspoon ground black pepper
- 1 1/2 teaspoons garlic powder
- 3 tablespoons Worcestershire sauce
- 2 tablespoons Dijon mustard
- 3 tablespoons grated Parmesan

- 2 tablespoons creamy vinaigrette
- 1 tablespoon olive oil

Directions:

Combine salmon, breadcrumbs, parsley, eggs, green onions, seafood herbs, black pepper, garlic powder, Worcestershire sauce, parmesan cheese, Dijon mustard, and creamy vinaigrette; divide and shape into eight patties.

Heat olive oil in a large frying pan over medium heat. Bake the salmon patties in portions until golden brown, 5 to 7 minutes per side. Repeat if necessary, with more olive oil.

Nutrition:

263 calories

12.3 g fat

10.8 g of carbohydrates

27.8 g of protein

95 mg cholesterol

782 mg of sodium

25.   Cajun Seafood Pasta

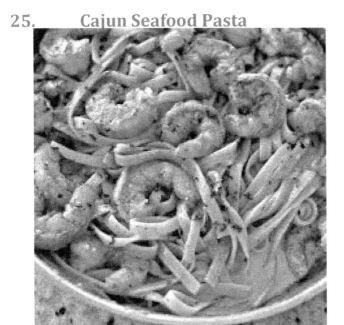

Preparation Time: 15 minutes

Cooking Time: 16 minutes

Servings: 2

Ingredients:

- 2 cups thick whipped cream
- 1 tablespoon chopped fresh basil
- 1 tablespoon chopped fresh thyme
- 2 teaspoons salt
- 2 teaspoons ground black pepper
- 1 1/2 teaspoon ground red pepper flakes
- 1 teaspoon ground white pepper
- 1 cup chopped green onions

- 1 cup chopped parsley
- 1/2 shrimp, peeled
- 1/2 cup scallops
- 1/2 cup of grated Swiss cheese
- 1/2 cup grated Parmesan cheese
- 1-pound dry fettuccine pasta

Directions:

Cook the pasta in a large pot with boiling salted water until al dente.

Meanwhile, pour the cream into a large skillet. Cook over medium heat, constantly stirring until it boils. Reduce heat and add spices, salt, pepper, onions, and parsley. Let simmer for 7 to 8 minutes or until thick.

Stir seafood and cook until shrimp are no longer transparent. Stir in the cheese and mix well.

Drain the pasta. Serve the sauce over the noodles.

Nutrition:

695 calories

36.7 grams of fat

62.2 g carbohydrates

31.5 g of protein

193 mg cholesterol

1054 mg of sodium

26.   Seafood Enchiladas

Preparation Time: 15 minutes

Cooking Time: 30 minutes

Servings: 2

Ingredients:

- 1 onion, minced
- 1 tablespoon butter
- 1/2 pound of fresh crab meat
- 1/4-pound shrimp - peeled, gutted and coarsely chopped
- 8 grams of Colby cheese
- 6 flour tortillas (10 inches)
- 1 cup half and half cream
- 1/2 cup sour cream
- 1/4 cup melted butter
- 1 1/2 teaspoon dried parsley
- 1/2 teaspoon garlic salt

Directions:

Preheat the oven to 175 ° C (350 ° F).

Fry the onions in a large frying pan in 1 tablespoon butter until they are transparent. Remove the pan from the heat and stir in the crab meat and shrimp. Grate the cheese and mix half of the seafood.

Place a large spoon of the mixture in each tortilla. Roll the tortillas around the mixture and place them in a 9 x 13-inch baking dish.

In a saucepan over medium heat, combine half and half, sour cream, 1/4 cup butter, parsley and garlic salt. Stir until the mixture is lukewarm and mixed. Pour the sauce over the enchiladas and sprinkle with the remaining cheese.

Bake in the preheated oven for 30 minutes.

Nutrition:

607 calories

36.5 grams of fat

42.6 g carbohydrates

26.8 g of protein

136 mg of cholesterol

1078 mg of sodium

27.   Easy Tuna Patties

Preparation Time: 15 minutes

Cooking Time: 10 minutes

Servings: 2

Ingredients:

- 2 teaspoons lemon juice
- 3 tablespoons grated Parmesan
- 2 eggs
- 10 tablespoons Italian breadcrumbs
- 3 tuna cans, drained
- 3 tablespoons diced onion
- 1 pinch of ground black pepper
- 3 tablespoons vegetable oil

Directions:

Beat the eggs and lemon juice in a bowl. Stir in the Parmesan cheese and breadcrumbs to obtain a paste. Add tuna and onion until everything is well mixed. Season with black pepper. Form the tuna mixture into eight 1-inch-thick patties.

Heat the vegetable oil in a frying pan over medium heat; fry the patties until golden brown, about 5 minutes on each side.

Nutrition:

325 calories

15.5 grams of fat

13.9 g of carbohydrates

31.3 g of protein

125 mg cholesterol

409 mg of sodium

28.   Fish Tacos

Preparation Time: 40 minutes

Cooking Time: 15 minutes

Servings: 2

Ingredients:

- 1 cup flour
- 2 tablespoons corn flour
- 1 teaspoon baking powder
- 1/2 teaspoon of salt
- 1 egg
- 1 cup of beer
- 1/2 cup of yogurt
- 1/2 cup of mayonnaise
- 1 lime, juice
- 1 jalapeño pepper, minced
- 1 c. Finely chopped capers
- 1/2 teaspoon dried oregano
- 1/2 teaspoon ground cumin
- 1/2 teaspoon dried dill
- 1 teaspoon ground cayenne pepper
- 1 liter of oil for frying
- 1 pound of cod fillets, 2-3 ounces each
- 8 corn tortillas
- 1/2 medium cabbage, finely shredded

Directions:

Prepare beer dough: combine flour, corn flour, baking powder and salt in a large bowl. Mix the egg and the beer and stir in the flour mixture quickly.

To make a white sauce: combine yogurt and mayonnaise in a medium bowl. Gradually add fresh lime juice until it is slightly fluid — season with jalapeño, capers, oregano, cumin, dill, and cayenne pepper.

Heat the oil in a frying pan.

Lightly sprinkle the fish with flour. Dip it in the beer batter and fry until crispy and golden brown. Drain on kitchen paper. Heat the tortillas. Place the fried fish in a tortilla and garnish with grated cabbage and white sauce.

Nutrition:

409 calories

18.8 g of fat

43 grams of carbohydrates

17.3 g of protein

54 mg cholesterol

407 mg of sodium

29.   Blackened Salmon Fillets

Preparation Time: 15 minutes

Cooking Time: 10 minutes

Servings: 2

Ingredients:

- 2 tablespoons paprika powder
- 1 tablespoon cayenne pepper powder
- 1 tablespoon onion powder
- 2 teaspoons salt
- 1/2 teaspoon ground white pepper
- 1/2 teaspoon ground black pepper
- 1/4 teaspoon dried thyme
- 1/4 teaspoon dried basil
- 1/4 teaspoon dried oregano
- 4 salmon fillets, skin and bones removed
- 1/2 cup unsalted butter, melted

Directions:

Combine bell pepper, cayenne pepper, onion powder, salt, white pepper, black pepper, thyme, basil and oregano in a small bowl.

Brush salmon fillets with 1/4 cup butter and sprinkle evenly with the cayenne pepper mixture. Sprinkle each fillet with ½ of the remaining butter.

Cook the salmon in a large heavy-bottomed pan, until dark, 2 to 5 minutes. Turn the fillets, sprinkle with the remaining butter and continue to cook until the fish easily peels with a fork.

Nutrition:

511 calories

38.3 grams of fat

4.5 grams of carbohydrates

37.4 g of protein

166 mg cholesterol

1248 mg of sodium

30. Brown Butter Perch

Preparation Time: 15 minutes

Cooking Time: 10 minutes

Servings: 2

Ingredients:

- 1 cup flour
- 1 teaspoon salt
- 1/2 teaspoon finely ground black pepper
- 1/2 teaspoon cayenne pepper
- 8 oz. fresh perch fillets
- 2 tablespoons butter
- 1 lemon cut in half

Directions:

In a bowl, beat flour, salt, black pepper, and cayenne pepper. Gently squeeze the perch fillets into the flour mixture to coat well and remove excess flour.

Heat the butter in a frying pan over medium heat until it is foamy and brown hazel. Place the fillets in portions in the pan and cook them light brown, about 2 minutes on each side. Place the cooked fillets on a plate, squeeze the lemon juice, and serve.

Nutrition:

271 calories

11.5 g of fat

30.9 g of carbohydrates

12.6 g of protein

43 mg of cholesterol

703 mg of sodium

Dinner

31.　　Dill Chutney Salmon

Preparation Time: 5 minutes

Cooking Time: 3 minutes

Servings: 2

Ingredients:

Chutney:

- ¼ cup fresh dill
- ¼ cup extra virgin olive oil
- Juice from ½ lemon
- Sea salt, to taste

Fish:

- 2 cups water
- 2 salmon fillets
- Juice from ½ lemon
- ¼ teaspoon paprika
- Salt and freshly ground pepper to taste

Directions:

Pulse all the chutney ingredients in a food processor until creamy. Set aside.

Add the water and steamer basket to the Instant Pot. Place salmon fillets, skin-side down, on the steamer basket. Drizzle the lemon juice over salmon and sprinkle with the paprika.

Secure the lid. Select the Manual mode and set the cooking time for 3 minutes at High Pressure.

Once cooking is complete, do a quick pressure release. Carefully open the lid.

Season the fillets with pepper and salt to taste. Serve topped with the dill chutney.

Nutrition:

Calories 636,

41g fat,

65g protein

32.   Garlic-Butter Parmesan Salmon and Asparagus

Preparation Time: 10 minutes

Cooking Time: 15 minutes

Servings: 2

Ingredients:

- 2 (6-ounce / 170-g) salmon fillets, skin on and patted dry
- Pink Himalayan salt
- Freshly ground black pepper, to taste
- 1 pound (454 g) fresh asparagus, ends snapped off
- 3 tablespoons almond butter
- 2 garlic cloves, minced
- ¼ cup grated Parmesan cheese

Directions:

Prep oven to 400ºF (205ºC). Line a baking sheet with aluminum foil.

Season both sides of the salmon fillets.

Situate salmon in the middle of the baking sheet and arrange the asparagus around the salmon.

Heat the almond butter in a small saucepan over medium heat.

Cook minced garlic

Drizzle the garlic-butter sauce over the salmon and asparagus and scatter the Parmesan cheese on top.

Bake in the preheated oven for about 12 minutes. You can switch the oven to broil at the end of cooking time for about 3 minutes to get a nice char on the asparagus.

Let cool for 5 minutes before serving.

Nutrition:

Calories 435,

26g fat,

42g protein

33.   Lemon Rosemary Roasted Branzino

Preparation Time: 15 minutes

Cooking Time: 30 minutes

Servings: 2

Ingredients:

- 4 tablespoons extra-virgin olive oil, divided
- 2 (8-ounce) Branzino fillets
- 1 garlic clove, minced
- 1 bunch scallions
- 10 to 12 small cherry tomatoes, halved
- 1 large carrot, cut into ¼-inch rounds
- ½ cup dry white wine
- 2 tablespoons paprika
- 2 teaspoons kosher salt
- ½ tablespoon ground chili pepper
- 2 rosemary sprigs or 1 tablespoon dried rosemary
- 1 small lemon, thinly sliced
- ½ cup sliced pitted kalamata olives

Directions:

Heat a large ovenproof skillet over high heat until hot, about 2 minutes. Add 1 tablespoon of olive oil and heat

Add the Branzino fillets, skin-side up, and sear for 2 minutes. Flip the fillets and cook. Set aside.

Swirl 2 tablespoons of olive oil around the skillet to coat evenly.

Add the garlic, scallions, tomatoes, and carrot, and sauté for 5 minutes

Add the wine, stirring until all ingredients are well combined. Carefully place the fish over the sauce.

Preheat the oven to 450ºF (235ºC).

Brush the fillets with the remaining 1 tablespoon of olive oil and season with paprika, salt, and chili pepper. Top each fillet with a rosemary sprig and lemon slices. Scatter the olives over fish and around the skillet.

Roast for about 10 minutes until the lemon slices are browned. Serve hot.

Nutrition:

Calories 724,

43g fat,

57g protein

34.   Grilled Lemon Pesto Salmon

Preparation Time: 5 minutes

Cooking Time: 10 minutes

Servings: 2

Ingredients:

- 10 ounces (283 g) salmon fillet
- 2 tablespoons prepared pesto sauce
- 1 large fresh lemon, sliced
- Cooking spray

Directions:

Preheat the grill to medium-high heat. Spray the grill grates with cooking spray.

Season the salmon well. Spread the pesto sauce on top.

Make a bed of fresh lemon slices about the same size as the salmon fillet on the hot grill, and place the salmon on top of the lemon slices. Put any additional lemon slices on top of the salmon.

Grill the salmon for 10 minutes.

Serve hot.

Nutrition:

Calories 316, 21g fat, 29g protein

35.   Steamed Trout with Lemon Herb Crust

Preparation Time: 10 minutes

Cooking Time: 15 minutes

Servings: 2

Ingredients:

- 3 tablespoons olive oil
- 3 garlic cloves, chopped
- 2 tablespoons fresh lemon juice
- 1 tablespoon chopped fresh mint
- 1 tablespoon chopped fresh parsley
- ¼ teaspoon dried ground thyme
- 1 teaspoon sea salt
- 1 pound (454 g) fresh trout (2 pieces)
- 2 cups fish stock

Directions:

Blend olive oil, garlic, lemon juice, mint, parsley, thyme, and salt. Brush the marinade onto the fish.

Insert a trivet in the Instant Pot. Fill in the fish stock and place the fish on the trivet.

Secure the lid. Select the Steam mode and set the cooking time for 15 minutes at High Pressure.

Once cooking is complete, do a quick pressure release. Carefully open the lid. Serve warm.

Nutrition:

Calories 477,

30g fat,

52g protein

36.   Roasted Trout Stuffed with Veggies

Preparation Time: 10 minutes

Cooking Time: 25 minutes

Servings: 2

Ingredient:

- 2 (8-ounce) whole trout fillets
- 1 tablespoon extra-virgin olive oil
- ¼ teaspoon salt
- 1/8 teaspoon black pepper
- 1 small onion, thinly sliced
- ½ red bell pepper
- 1 poblano pepper
- 2 or 3 shiitake mushrooms, sliced
- 1 lemon, sliced

Directions:

Set oven to 425ºF (220ºC). Coat baking sheet with nonstick cooking spray.

Rub both trout fillets, inside and out, with the olive oil. Season with salt and pepper.

Mix together the onion, bell pepper, poblano pepper, and mushrooms in a large bowl. Stuff half of this mix into the cavity of each fillet. Top the mixture with 2 or 3 lemon slices inside each fillet.

Place the fish on the prepared baking sheet side by side. Roast in the preheated oven for 25 minutes

Pullout from the oven and serve on a plate.

Nutrition:

Calories 453,

22g fat,

49g protein

37. Lemony Trout with Caramelized Shallots

Preparation Time: 10 minutes

Cooking Time: 20 minutes

Servings: 2

Ingredients:

- Shallots:
- 1 teaspoon almond butter
- 2 shallots, thinly sliced
- Dash salt
- Trout:
- 1 tablespoon almond butter
- 2 (4-ounce / 113-g) trout fillets
- 3 tablespoons capers
- ¼ cup freshly squeezed lemon juice
- ¼ teaspoon salt
- Dash freshly ground black pepper
- 1 lemon, thinly sliced

Directions:

For Shallots

Situate skillet over medium heat, cook the butter, shallots, and salt for 20 minutes, stirring every 5 minutes.

For Trout

Meanwhile, in another large skillet over medium heat, heat 1 teaspoon of almond butter.

Add the trout fillets and cook each side for 3 minutes, or until flaky. Transfer to a plate and set aside.

In the skillet used for the trout, stir in the capers, lemon juice, salt, and pepper, then bring to a simmer. Whisk in the remaining 1 tablespoon of almond butter. Spoon the sauce over the fish.

Garnish the fish with the lemon slices and caramelized shallots before serving.

Nutrition:

Calories 344,

18g fat,

21g protein

38.   Easy Tomato Tuna Melts

Preparation Time: 5 minutes

Cooking Time: 4 minutes

Servings: 2

Ingredients:

- 1 (5-oz) can chunk light tuna packed in water
- 2 tablespoons plain Greek yogurt
- 2 tablespoons finely chopped celery
- 1 tablespoon finely chopped red onion
- 2 teaspoons freshly squeezed lemon juice
- 1 large tomato, cut into ¾-inch-thick rounds
- ½ cup shredded Cheddar cheese

Directions:

Preheat the broiler to High.

Stir together the tuna, yogurt, celery, red onion, lemon juice, and cayenne pepper in a medium bowl.

Place the tomato rounds on a baking sheet. Top each with some tuna salad and Cheddar cheese.

Broil for 3 to 4 minutes until the cheese is melted and bubbly. Cool for 5 minutes before serving.

Nutrition:

Calories 244, 10g fat, 30g protein

39.   Mackerel and Green Bean Salad

Preparation Time: 10 minutes

Cooking Time: 10 minutes

Servings: 2

Ingredients:

- 2 cups green beans
- 1 tablespoon avocado oil
- 2 mackerel fillets
- 4 cups mixed salad greens
- 2 hard-boiled eggs, sliced
- 1 avocado, sliced
- 2 tablespoons lemon juice
- 2 tablespoons olive oil
- 1 teaspoon Dijon mustard
- Salt and black pepper, to taste

Directions:

Cook the green beans in pot of boiling water for about 3 minutes. Drain and set aside.

Melt the avocado oil in a pan over medium heat. Add the mackerel fillets and cook each side for 4 minutes.

Divide the greens between two salad bowls. Top with the mackerel, sliced egg, and avocado slices.

Scourge lemon juice, olive oil, mustard, salt, and pepper, and drizzle over the salad. Add the cooked green beans and toss to combine, then serve.

Nutrition:

Calories 737,

57g fat,

34g protein

40.   Hazelnut Crusted Sea Bass

Preparation Time: 10 minutes

Cooking Time: 15 minutes

Servings: 2

Ingredients:

- 2 tablespoons almond butter
- 2 sea bass fillets
- 1/3 cup roasted hazelnuts
- A pinch of cayenne pepper

Direction

Ready oven to 425ºF (220ºC). Line a baking dish with waxed paper.

Brush the almond butter over the fillets.

Pulse the hazelnuts and cayenne in a food processor. Coat the sea bass with the hazelnut mixture, then transfer to the baking dish.

Bake in the preheated oven for about 15 minutes. Cool for 5 minutes before serving.

Nutrition:

Calories 468,

31g fat,

40g protein

Dessert

41.   Feta Cheesecake

Preparation Time: 30 Minutes

Cooking Time: 90 Minutes

Servings: 12

Ingredients:

- 2 cups graham cracker crumbs (about 30 crackers)
- ½ tsp ground cinnamon
- 6 tbsps. unsalted butter, melted
- ½ cup sesame seeds, toasted
- 12 ounces cream cheese, softened
- 1 cup crumbled feta cheese
- 3 large eggs
- 1 cup of sugar
- 2 cups plain yogurt
- 2 tbsps. grated lemon zest
- 1 tsp vanilla

Directions:

Set the oven to 350°F.

Mix the cracker crumbs, butter, cinnamon, and sesame seeds with a fork. Move the combination to a springform pan and spread until it is even. Refrigerate.

In a separate bowl, mix the cream cheese and feta. With an electric mixer, beat both kinds of cheese together. Add the eggs one after the other, beating the mixture with each new addition. Add sugar, then keep beating until creamy. Mix in yogurt, vanilla, and lemon zest.

Bring out the refrigerated springform and spread the batter on it. Then place it in a baking pan. Pour water in the pan till it is halfway full.

Bake for about 50 minutes. Remove cheesecake and allow it to cool. Refrigerate for at least 4 hours.

It is done. Serve when ready.

Nutrition:

Calories: 98kcal

Carbs: 7g

Fat: 7g

Protein: 3g

42.   Pear Croustade

Preparation Time: 30 Minutes

Cooking Time: 60 Minutes

Servings: 10

Ingredients:

- 1 cup plus 1 tbsp. all-purpose flour, divided
- 4 ½ tbsps. Sugar, divided
- 1/8 tsp salt
- 6 tbsps. Unsalted butter, chilled, cut into ½ inch cubes
- 1 large-sized egg, separated
- 1 ½ tbsps. Ice-cold water
- 3 firm, ripe pears (Bosc), peeled, cored, sliced into ¼ inch slices 1 tbsp. fresh lemon juice
- 1/3 tsp ground allspice
- 1 tsp anise seeds

Directions:

Pour 1 cup of flour, 1 ½ Tbsps. Of sugar, butter, and salt into a food processor and combine the ingredients by pulsing.

Whisk the yolk of the egg and ice water in a separate bowl. Mix the egg mixture with the flour mixture. It will form a dough, wrap it, and set aside for an hour.

Set the oven to 400°F.

Mix the pear, sugar, leftover flour, allspice, anise seed, and lemon juice in a large bowl to make a filling.

Arrange the filling on the center of the dough.

Bake for about 40 minutes. Cool for about 15 minutes before serving.

Nutrition:

Calories: 498kcal

Carbs: 32g

Fat: 32g

Protein: 18g

43.   Melomakarona

Preparation Time: 20 Minutes

Cooking Time: 45 Minutes

Servings: 20

Ingredients:

- 4 cups of sugar, divided
- 4 cups of water
- 1 cup plus 1 tbsp. honey, divided
- 1 (2-inch) strip orange peel, pith removed
- 1 cinnamon stick
- ½ cup extra-virgin olive oil
- ¼ cup unsalted butter,
- ¼ cup Metaxa brandy or any other brandy
- 1 tbsp. grated

Orange zest

- ¾ cup of orange juice
- ¼ tsp baking soda
- 3 cups pastry flour
- ¾ cup fine semolina flour
- 1 ½ tsp baking powder
- 4 tsp ground cinnamon, divided
- 1 tsp ground cloves, divided
- 1 cup finely chopped walnut
- 1/3 cup brown sugar

Directions:

Mix 3 ½ cups of sugar, 1 cup honey, orange peel, cinnamon stick, and water in a pot and heat it for about 10 minutes.

Mix the sugar, oil, and butter for about minutes, then add the brandy, leftover honey, and zest. Then add a mixture of baking soda and orange juice. Mix thoroughly.

In a distinct bowl, blend the pastry flour, baking powder, semolina, 2 tsp of cinnamon, and ½ tsp. of cloves. Add the mixture to the mixer slowly. Run the mixer until the ingredients form a dough. Cover and set aside for 30 minutes.

Set the oven to 350°F

With your palms, form small oval balls from the dough. Make a total of forty balls.

Bake the cookie balls for 30 minutes, then drop them in the prepared syrup.

Create a mixture with the walnuts, leftover cinnamon, and cloves. Spread the mixture on the top of the baked cookies.

Serve the cookies or store them in a closed-lid container.

Nutrition:

Calories: 294kcal

Carbs: 44g

Fat: 12g

Protein: 3g

44. Loukoumades (Fried Honey Balls)

Preparation Time: 20 Minutes

Cooking Time: 45 Minutes

Servings: 10

Ingredients:

- 2 cups of sugar
- 1 cup of water
- 1 cup honey
- 1 ½ cups tepid water
- 1 tbsp. brown sugar
- ¼ cup of vegetable oil
- 1 tbsp. active dry yeast
- 1 ½ cups all-purpose flour, 1 cup cornstarch, ½ tsp salt
- Vegetable oil for frying
- 1 ½ cups chopped walnuts
- ¼ cup ground cinnamon

Directions:

Boil the sugar and water on medium heat. Add honey after 10 minutes. cool and set aside.

Mix the tepid water, oil, brown sugar,' and yeast in a large bowl. Allow it to sit for 10 minutes. In a distinct bowl, blend the flour, salt, and cornstarch. With your hands mix the yeast and the flour to make a wet dough. Cover and set aside for 2 hours.

Fry in oil at 350°F. Use your palm to measure the sizes of the dough as they are dropped in the frying pan. Fry each batch for about 3-4 minutes.

Immediately the loukoumades are done frying, drop them in the prepared syrup.

Serve with cinnamon and walnuts.

Nutrition:

Calories: 355kcal

Carbs: 64g

Fat: 7g

Protein: 6g

45.   Crème Caramel

Preparation Time: 60 Minutes

Cooking Time: 60 Minutes

Servings: 12

Ingredients:

- 5 cups of whole milk
- 2 tsp vanilla extract
- 8 large egg yolks
- 4 large-sized eggs
- 2 cups sugar, divided
- ¼ cup 0f water

Directions:

Preheat the oven to 350°F

Heat the milk with medium heat wait for it to be scalded.

Mix 1 cup of sugar and eggs in a bowl and add it to the eggs.

With a nonstick pan on high heat, boil the water and remaining sugar. Do not stir, instead whirl the pan. When the sugar forms caramel, divide it into ramekins.

Divide the egg mixture into the ramekins and place in a baking pan. Increase water to the pan until it is half full. Bake for 30 minutes.

Remove the ramekins from the baking pan, cool, then refrigerate for at least 8 hours.

Serve.

Nutrition:

Calories: 110kcal

Carbs: 21g

Fat: 1g

Protein: 2g

46.   Galaktoboureko

Preparation Time: 30 Minutes

Cooking Time: 90 Minutes

Servings: 12

Ingredients:

- 4 cups sugar, divided
- 1 tbsp. fresh lemon juice
- 1 cup of water
- 1 Tbsp. plus 1 ½ tsp grated lemon zest, divided into 10 cups
- Room temperature whole milk
- 1 cup plus 2 tbsps. unsalted butter, melted and divided into 2
- Tbsps. vanilla extract
- 7 large-sized eggs
- 1 cup of fine semolina
- 1 package phyllo, thawed and at room temperature

Directions:

Preheat oven to 350°F

Mix 2 cups of sugar, lemon juice, 1 ½ tsp of lemon zest, and water. Boil over medium heat. Set aside.

Mix the milk, 2 Tbsps. of butter, and vanilla in a pot and put-on medium heat. Remove from heat when milk is scalded

Mix the eggs and semolina in a bowl, then add the mixture to the scalded milk. Put the egg-milk mixture on medium heat. Stir until it forms a custard-like material.

Brush butter on each sheet then arrange all over the baking pan until everywhere is covered. Spread the custard on the bottom pile phyllo

Arrange the buttered phyllo all over the top of the custard until every inch is covered.

Bake for about 40 minutes. cover the top of the pie with all the prepared syrup. Serve.

Nutrition:

Calories: 393kcal

Carbs: 55g

Fat: 15g

Protein: 8g

47. Kourabiedes Almond Cookies

Preparation Time: 20 Minutes

Cooking Time: 50 Minutes

Servings: 20

Ingredients:

- 1 ½ cups unsalted butter, clarified, at room temperature 2 cups
- Confectioners' sugar, divided
- 1 large egg yolk
- 2 tbsps. brandy
- 1 1/2 tsp baking powder
- 1 tsp vanilla extract
- 5 cups all-purpose flour, sifted
- 1 cup roasted almonds, chopped

Directions:

Preheat the oven to 350°F

Thoroughly mix butter and ½ cup of sugar in a bowl. Add in the egg after a while. Create a brandy mixture by mixing the brandy and baking powder. Add the mixture to the egg, add vanilla, then keep beating until the ingredients are properly blended

Add flour and almonds to make a dough.

Roll the dough to form crescent shapes. You should be able to get about 40 pieces. Place the pieces on a baking sheet, then bake in the oven for 25 minutes.

Allow the cookies to cool, then coat them with the remaining confectioner's sugar.

Serve.

Nutrition:

Calories: 102kcal

Carbs: 10g

Fat: 7g

Protein: 2g

48.   Ekmek Kataifi

Preparation Time: 30 Minutes

Cooking Time: 45 Minutes

Servings: 10

Ingredients:

- 1 cup of sugar
- 1 cup of water
- 2 (2-inch) strips lemon peel, pith removed
- 1 tbsp. fresh lemon juice
- ½ cup plus 1 tbsp. unsalted butter, melted
- ½lbs. frozen kataifi pastry, thawed, at room temperature
- 2 ½ cups whole milk
- ½ tsp. ground mastiha
- 2 large eggs
- ¼ cup fine semolina
- 1 tsp. of cornstarch
- ¼ cup of sugar
- ½ cup sweetened coconut flakes
- 1 cup whipping cream
- 1 tsp. vanilla extract
- 1 tsp. powdered milk
- 3 tbsps. of confectioners' sugar
- ½ cup chopped unsalted pistachios

Directions:

Set the oven to 350°F. Grease the baking pan with 1. Tbsp of butter.

Put a pot on medium heat, then add water, sugar, lemon juice, lemon peel. Leave to boil for about 10 minutes. Reserve.

Untangle the kataifi, coat with the leftover butter, then place in the baking pan.

Mix the milk and mastiha, then place it on medium heat. Remove from heat when the milk is scalded, then cool the mixture.

Mix the eggs, cornstarch, semolina, and sugar in a bowl, stir thoroughly, then whisk the cooled milk mixture into the bowl.

Transfer the egg and milk mixture to a pot and place on heat. Wait for it to thicken like custard, then add the coconut flakes and cover it with a plastic wrap. Cool.

Spread the cooled custard-like material over the kataifi. Place in the refrigerator for at least 8 hours.

Strategically remove the kataifi from the pan with a knife. Take it away in such a way that the mold faces up.

Whip a cup of cream, add 1 tsp. vanilla, 1tsp. powdered milk, and 3 tbsps. Of sugar. Spread the mixture all over the custard, wait for it to harden, then flip and add the leftover cream mixture to the kataifi side.

Serve.

Nutrition: Calories: 649kcal; Carbs: 37g; Fat: 52g; Protein: 11g

49.   Revani Syrup Cake

Preparation Time: 30 Minutes

Cooking Time: 3 Hours

Servings: 24

Ingredients:

- 1 tbsp. unsalted butter
- 2 tbsps. all-purpose flour
- 1 cup ground rusk or bread crumbs
- 1 cup fine semolina flour
- ¾ cup ground toasted almonds
- 3 tsp baking powder
- 16 large eggs
- 2 tbsps. vanilla extract
- 3 cups of sugar, divided
- 3 cups of water
- 5 (2-inch) strips lemon peel, pith removed
- 3 tbsps. fresh lemon juice
- 1 oz of brandy

Directions:

Preheat the oven to 350°F. Grease the baking pan with 1 Tbsp. of butter and flour.

Mix the rusk, almonds, semolina, baking powder in a bowl.

In another bowl, mix the eggs, 1 cup of sugar, vanilla, and whisk with an electric mixer for about 5 minutes. Add the semolina mixture to the eggs and stir.

Pour the stirred batter into the greased baking pan and place in the preheated oven.

With the remaining sugar, lemon peels, and water make the syrup by boiling the mixture on medium heat. Add the lemon juice after 6 minutes, then cook for 3 minutes. Remove the lemon peels and set the syrup aside.

After the cake is done in the oven, spread the syrup over the cake.

Cut the cake as you please and serve.

Nutrition:

Calories: 348kcal

Carbs: 55g

Fat: 9g

Protein: 5g

50.   Almonds and Oats Pudding

Preparation Time: 10 Minutes

Cooking Time: 15 Minutes

Servings: 4

Ingredients:

- 1 tablespoon lemon juice
- Zest of 1 lime
- 1 and ½ cups of almond milk
- 1 teaspoon almond extract
- ½ cup oats
- 2 tablespoons stevia
- ½ cup silver almonds, chopped

Directions:

In a pan, blend the almond milk plus the lime zest and the other ingredients, whisk, bring to a simmer and cook over medium heat for 15 minutes.

Split the mix into bowls then serve cold.

Nutrition:

Calories 174

Fat 12.1

Fiber 3.2

Carbs 3.9

Protein 4.8

Conclusion

Again, thanks for purchasing this book.

Here are some commonly asked questions about Mediterranean Diet and you, yourself, might be one of the individuals who have something troubling their mind about this diet.

1. What's the Main Idea behind the Mediterranean Diet?

The main concept behind this diet is a simple one. The idea is to model the diet after the people of the Mediterranean who eat simple, natural foods. Their dietary habits have been shown to increase lifespan, lose weight, lower the rates of heart disease and cancer, along with a bevy of other diseases like lowering the odds of Alzheimer's or Parkinson's.

2. Who Should I Consult Before I Start on The Mediterranean Diet?

You should always consult a doctor, physician, or a dietitian before starting any new type of meal plan or diet. You want someone who can give you the right information based on what is right for your specific set of needs.

3. Do I Need to Drink Wine on This Diet? What Is the Recommended Amount I Should Have Daily?

Women should consume approximately 2.5% of calories from wine on this diet. Men should consume approximately 5% of calories from wine. That being said, wine is a completely optional part of this diet and is not necessary for it to be effective.

4. What Is an Aromatic Olive Oil?

Aromatic olive oil has been made in Greece for as long as it can be remembered. This type of oil has herbs and spices added to it. Aromatic olive oil is known throughout the world for its antioxidant, astringent, and medicinal properties. Herbs supply the antioxidant properties to the olive oil and prevent oxidation. It also helps to improve the flavor which is a nice added bonus.

The different ingredients of aromatic olive oil are listed below:

Spices: Cardamom, Cedar Fruit, Coriander, Cumin Seed, Nutmeg, Aniseed, Ginger, Guinea Grains, Cinnamon, Pepper, and Fennel Seed.

Herbs and Aromatic Plants: Lay, Marjoram, Oregano, Basil, Mint, Spearmint, Sage, Rosemary, Thyme, Tarragon, Savory, Parsley, Fresh Fennel, Dill, and Coriander.

Vegetables: Garlic, Red Hot Peppers, Sun-Dried Tomatoes, Red Sweet Peppers, Capers, Truffles, and Chinese Mushrooms.

5. What Health Benefits Are Directly Associated with The Mediterranean Diet?

Studies have shown that the Mediterranean diet is associated with prolonged longevity, overall greater health, lower rates of cancers (particularly breast, colon, uterus, and prostate), and a lower rate of cardiovascular disease. These benefits are attributed to the diet composition and the active Mediterranean lifestyle.

7. What Type of Effect Does the Mediterranean Diet Have in Lowering One's Chance of Heart Disease?

Studies have shown this diet plays an important role in lowering heart disease. This is due to the fact that the Mediterranean diet promotes a more holistic approach to eating and staying healthy. Another factor is the inclusion of red wine as part of the diet. Red wine has been shown to lower the odds of heart disease when consumed in moderate amounts.

8. What Role Does Exercise Play in The Mediterranean Diet?

The Mediterranean diet was developed in the 1960's. During this time physical activity and exercise was a regular part of the culture in the region of the Mediterranean. This is one of the main reasons why the Mediterranean diet emphasizes the importance of having a regular exercise routine to attain better health. I like to go on daily walks and I try to swim a few times each week. Make your exercise fun and you won't have a problem incorporating it into your daily routine.

9. What Is the Difference Between A Low-Carb Diet and The Mediterranean Diet?

The main difference between these types of diet is protein. Generally, the Mediterranean diet has lower protein content. On the Mediterranean diet, you only get approximately 15% of your daily calories from the protein. On low-carb diets, the majority of your daily calories comes in the form of protein.

10. What Is the Mediterranean Diet's View on The Fattening Foods It Recommends We Eat?

The Mediterranean diet promotes consuming foods like bread, pasta, nuts, and rice. All of these foods have been traditionally perceived as being fattening. While these foods do contain higher fat content than other types of food the Mediterranean diet preaches having them in moderation. These types of food are bulkier in nature and will make you feel more satisfied than foods that are refined or processed. Add in some vegetables and fruits to go along with these fattening foods and you'll feel satisfied quicker and for a longer period of time. Always be aware of what and how much you're putting in your body. The sooner you get good at this important step the better off you'll be.

Thanks, and Good Luck.

117

CPSIA information can be obtained
at www.ICGtesting.com
Printed in the USA
BVHW052349080421
604476BV00004B/1125